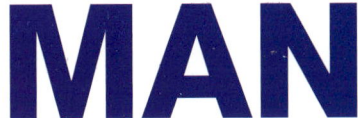

CONTENTS

Weighty matters	2
Getting active – and keeping your weight down	4
Coping with stress	6
Stopping smoking	10
Sensible drinking	12
Drugs and substance use	13
Eyes	14
Ears	15
Mouth matters	16
Back pain	17
Sexually transmitted infections (STIs)	20
Erectile dysfunction (ED, impotence)	21
Prostate problems	22
Bowel cancer	24
Skin cancer	26
Testicular cancer	28
When health problems develop	29
Getting the best from the NHS	30
Contacts	Rear cover

Introduction

As the proud owner of the latest Man model you will be keen to keep your bodywork in top condition. With a little care this high performance machine will last a long lifetime with minimal need for maintenance or spare parts. So with this manual you are more than just a standard model. You are more, much more. You are a highly-tuned Male #1 and you might just reach the finish-line without your original exhaust pipe falling off.

Weighty matters

Eating a well-balanced diet can improve your health by:
- Keeping your weight down
- Lowering your blood cholesterol
- Preventing high blood pressure.

All of these lower your risk of getting heart disease and help prevent things like diabetes and cancer.

See www.malehealth.co.uk/diet

> ### Fat facts
> You do need to eat a little fat because it helps the body soak up some vitamins, boosts energy and supplies some of the things the body can't make itself such as vitamins and building blocks for hormones. But too much fat means too much weight.
>
> - Look for foods that are lower in fat (check the label and go for fresh foods)
> - Fish and chips won't kill you, but eating high fat foods all the time can seriously damage your health
> - Cut down on the fat you use in cooking. Grill, casserole or stew meat instead of frying it.

Boring? I'll eat my hat

Eating well doesn't need to be boring. Eating a good variety of food makes sense and can be very tasty too. Basically you need:
- More fruit and vegetables
- Some starchy foods such as rice, bread, pasta and potatoes
- Less saturated fat, salt and sugar
- Some protein-rich foods such as fresh meat, fish, eggs and pulses

Salt and increased blood pressure

Eating too much salt can raise your blood pressure. People with high blood pressure are three times more likely to develop heart disease or have a stroke than people with normal blood pressure.

Tips to reduce salt
- Eat home-cooked meals rather than ready meals when possible
- Use fresh fish and lean meat, rather than canned, smoked or processed meat, helping to reduce fat as well
- Go for food with low or reduced sodium levels or no added salt
- Cook rice, pasta and hot cereals without salt
- Use herbs and spices instead of salt when cooking.

Fruit and veg

Unless you have been hiding under a rock for the past few years you will know that eating plenty of fruit and vegetables is good for your health. Aim to eat at least five portions a day.

Heavyweight issues

Did you know that:

- Men with waist sizes over 40 inches are 33% more likely to die from cancer than those who are a healthy weight?
- 2 out of every 5 people in the United Kingdom have high blood pressure which is often linked to being overweight?
- A person who is 12kg (about two stone) overweight is twice as likely to have a heart attack as someone who is a healthy weight?
- Every year, 30,000 deaths are directly linked to obesity, and every 17.5 minutes a person dies of an obesity-related illness?

Good gut size

Men with a waist size of more than 94 centimetres (37 inches) have increased health risks. A waist measurement of over 102 centimetres (40 inches) can lead to serious health risks.

African-Caribbean and Asian men have an increased risk of developing diabetes, high blood pressure and heart disease, and being overweight increases this risk. Being 40 years old is fine, having a 40-inch waist isn't.

How to measure your waist
- Find the top of your hip bone and the bottom of your ribs
- Breathe out naturally
- Place the tape measure between these points and wrap it around your waist
- Make a note of the measurement.

Body mass index (BMI)

- Measure your height in metres and your weight in kilograms;
- Divide your weight by your height squared = weight (kg) / height (m) x height (m);
- Make a note of the result (your BMI).

Normal BMI for an adult is 18.5 to 24.9. If your BMI is over 25 you should consider losing weight; a BMI of 30 or over is considered obese and you definitely need to lose weight.

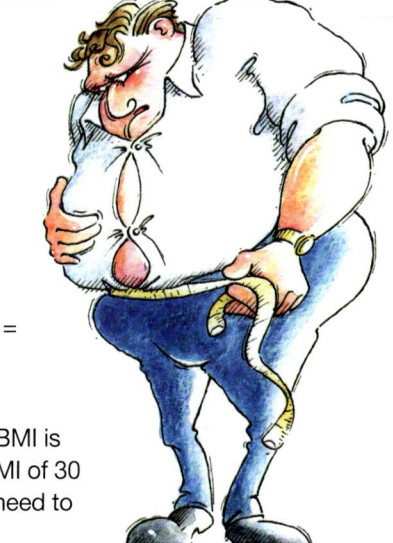

Getting active – and keeping your weight down

Even if you eat the correct foods and have a healthy balanced diet it is still important to be active and fit. Research shows that fitness is a strong measure of health and can lead to an improved quality of life. Being fit improves your overall health and reduces your risk of disease.

Activity

Around 100,000 UK men die every year before they reach even the age of 70. That's one man every 4½ minutes. Some men can run a mile in under that time.

Lack of physical activity together with poor diet has led to more than 1 in 5 men in England now being seriously overweight. A further 40% are overweight. Diabetes caused by obesity is increasing fast. Diabetes is one of the single most common causes of erectile dysfunction (ED or impotence). Being up for it may be a bigger problem than you think.

Routine maintenance

Men who increase their activity level over a five year period cut their chances of dying early by almost half. Walking instead of using the car helps your health, your bank balance and the environment. Exercise will make you feel better, make you look better and who knows… maybe even make you more attractive (showers permitting of course!).

Of course many jobs require lots of exercise. But if yours doesn't, there are simple things you can consider doing to make exercise part of your normal working day. And what better way to start than with the journey to work in the morning?

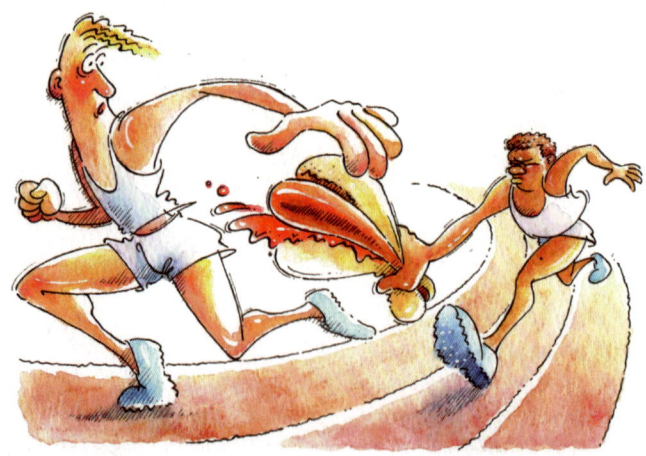

Travelling to and from work

The journey to work is an ideal chance to help build up the 30 minutes a day of regular physical activity you need. It also has added benefits, as you could save on petrol, fares and commuter stress.

Walking or cycling to work (or to the station if you have a longer journey), instead of driving or using public transport, could make a huge difference. If it takes you 15 minutes each way, you would immediately achieve your recommended daily amount of exercise – and it may even take less time than battling through the traffic.

If your employer doesn't already have schemes in place, ask if they can help to encourage walking and cycling to work.

At work

There are a number of simple things you can do during the work day to stay active – and remember the little things add up!

- Take the stairs instead of the lift; if you work on the top floor, get off a few floors early
- Take opportunities to walk around the office: deliver documents or messages to co-workers in person rather than by email
- Go for a walk at lunch time and during breaks
- Maybe join a sports team for lunchtime or after work.

The gym

If there is a gym attached to your workplace, you could use it before or after work, or during your lunch break. Otherwise you could ask whether your employer is willing to subsidise membership of an external gym or sports centre as both of you will benefit from your improved health and fitness.

Lack of physical activity together with poor diet has led to more than 1 in 5 men in England now being obese. A further 40% are overweight.

Your weight

Experts agree that in order to lose weight people should be active for up to 60 minutes at least three times a week, in addition to the 30 minutes of daily activity. This probably means taking up a sport or some other form of structured exercise – but it may also be possible to spend more time and push yourself harder in your everyday activities, such as walking to meetings at work, climbing stairs instead of using the lift – or doing more DIY in the evenings or at weekends.

The two main indicators of whether you need to lose weight are waist measurement, and body mass index (BMI) – see page 3.

Coping with stress

Pressure at work can be good for you, but if the experience of pressure is excessive or prolonged, you may begin to feel stressed.

Irrespective of the source of your stress, you should speak to your manager or someone else you feel comfortable talking to in your organisation. If it is work-related, your employer has a duty to take reasonable steps to try to resolve the problem. If it is not work-related they may be able to support you in some way or help to take some pressure off you at work while you resolve the stress in your personal life. Talking these things through is not a sign of weakness: It really can help.

> 5 million people of working age have a common mental health disorder, such as stress, depression, anxiety, addiction, etc. Over 40% of time off work is due to mental ill-health.

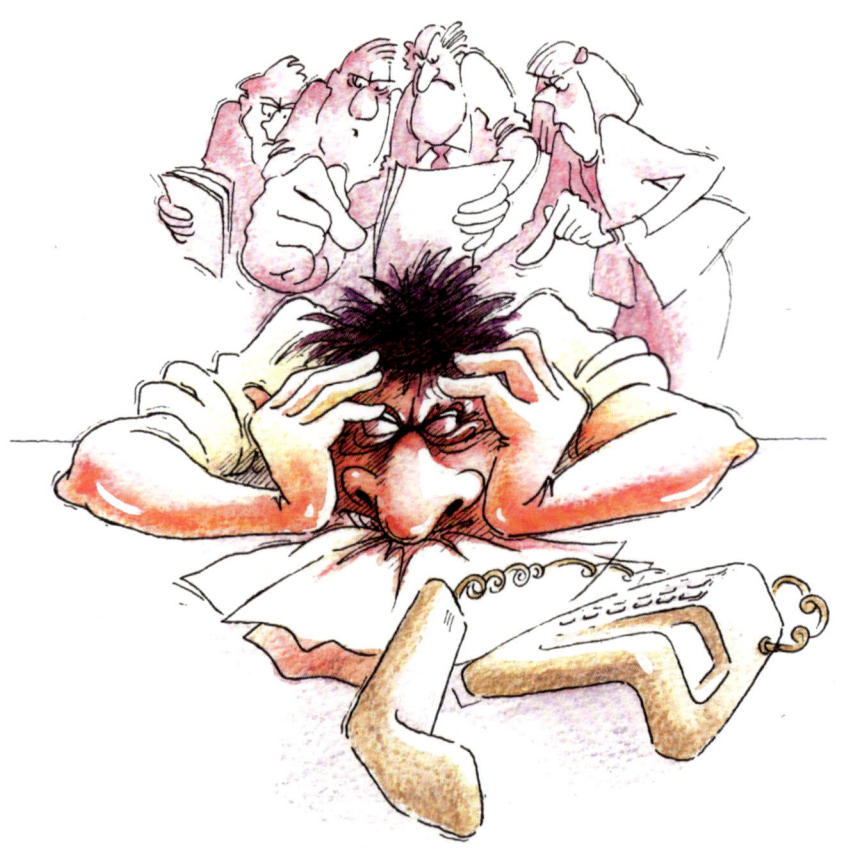

A relentless build-up of pressure, without the opportunity to recover, can lead to harmful stress. The important thing is to recognise the warning signs while you can do something about it.

Common signs are:
- Eating more or less than normal
- Mood swings
- Poor concentration
- Feeling tense or anxious
- Low self-esteem
- Not sleeping properly
- Tiredness
- Poor memory or forgetfulness
- Excessive drinking and/or drug use.

The good news is that there are positive steps that you can take to deal with and manage stress, both at home and at work. Our five top tips are …

1 Time out

It can be hard to be rational when you are feeling very stressed, which is why it's important to take some time out.

Quick fix
Physically removing yourself from a stressful situation, even for a few moments, can give you the space you need to feel more able to tackle the problem. If you anticipate a stressful day, try to get up a bit earlier to prepare for it instead of feeling rushed.

Long-term fix
Taking time out from your everyday routine may help you deal with, and avoid, stress. At work, try to avoid doing long hours and make sure you use your annual leave entitlement, plan your holidays and mini-breaks.

2 Work out

Exercise can help to prevent stress related ill-health.

Quick fix
Go for a quick walk round the block. This can help clear your head and put problems in perspective so you are able to tackle them with renewed energy. At work, get some fresh air and get moving during breaks.

Long-term fix
Aim to do at least 30 minutes of activity a day, as recommended to remain healthy. Regular activity may help reduce your stress levels as well as getting you fit and making you feel good.

3 Chill out

Making time for yourself mentally and emotionally, as well as getting enough quality sleep is important so you can focus on relaxing your mind and recharging.

Quick fix

Learning simple relaxation techniques can be an effective way of helping you deal with feelings of stress – try these simple exercises:

Deep breathing – take a long slow breath in through your nose (breathing-in from your belly), then very slowly breathe out through the mouth; really concentrate on your breathing, and after a few repetitions you should begin to feel more relaxed.

Tensing and stretching your muscles – rotate your neck to the side as far as is comfortable and then relax; repeat on the other side; then try fully tensing your shoulder and back muscles for several seconds, and then relax completely.

Long-term fix

Plan time to relax even if it's just having a long bath or listening to music. Try and have a good night's sleep – adults usually need, on average, 7 to 8 hours – and if this is not possible aim to have at least 4 hours of sleep at the same time each day as this can help to keep your sleep clock regular. Relaxation techniques or meditation can also be useful for many people in helping them to feel m ore able to cope – you can buy relaxation music, and there are many types of relaxation classes available like meditation, yoga and pilates.

> At any one time one worker in six will be experiencing depression, anxiety or problems relating to stress. Mental ill health is normal in every workplace in the land.

4 Leave it out

Try to avoid taking refuge in smoking, junk food or alcohol! This won't help your stress levels. Avoid too many caffeinated and sugary drinks as they may make you feel more anxious and bursts of sugar can cause mood swings.

Quick fix

Drink plenty of water. This will help you to concentrate better, and may stop you getting stress headaches which can be caused by dehydration.

Long-term fix

Improving your diet and drinking plenty of water will increase your body's resistance to stress. Eating fruit and vegetables really boosts your immune system, especially in times of stress. It's important to make time for proper meals to help you stay energised.

5 Talk it out

Talking about stress with family, friends or colleagues may help you see things in a different light and find a way forward in tackling the underlying problems.

You may also want to consider talking to a healthcare professional, such as your GP or practice nurse. If your organisation has a counselling or occupational health service, then use it. Research shows that people with work-based stress have benefitted from such services.

Finally, if you can't find a solution

You may need to highlight the problem with your boss and seek his/her support.

- Book a time with your boss to meet
- Prepare; consider what is causing you stress and any potential solutions you may have thought of
- Think about positive changes that you would like to make to help you work more effectively
- Make a list of points and questions that you want to cover
- Help your boss to help you by giving the information he/she needs
- Find out if there are any training courses (for example in time management or problem solving) that may help you cope better
- Arrange a follow-up meeting to make sure you and your boss are happy with how things are progressing
- If you don't want to speak direct to your boss, you could raise the issue with a staff or trade union representative who can then speak on your behalf.

Useful contacts

Health and Safety Executive
www.hse.gov.uk/stress

MIND (National Association for Mental Health)
0300 123 3393
www.mind.org.uk

Stopping smoking

Smoking is the single greatest cause of death in the developed world. It has killed more people than both world wars put together – and still kills 114,000 people each year in the UK, commonly through lung cancer and heart disease. One in ten moderate smokers and almost one in five heavy smokers (more than 15 cigarettes a day) will die of lung cancer.

> **Half of all smokers will die early!**

Smokers tend to develop coronary thrombosis (heart attacks) ten years earlier than non-smokers, and account for the vast majority of heart bypass patients. They also take 25% more sick days per year than non-smokers.

On a more positive note, the very moment you stop smoking your health will start to improve. After only 20 minutes of not smoking, your blood pressure and pulse return to normal. In just 48 hours, your body is nicotine-free and carbon monoxide is cleared from your system. And, within 2 to 12 weeks, your circulation improves and you feel noticeably fitter. Best of all, within 5 years your risk of lung cancer will have dropped dramatically, and your risk may be halved by the time you reach your 10th year of being cigarette-free.

Some people try to reduce their cigarette intake gradually. The trouble with this approach is that, as soon as something disturbs your concentration, the numbers tend to creep back up again. It's much better to stop.

Make sure you are ready to give up. Many fail because they jump into the task before they are ready. Have a 'quit plan' and make use of all the sources of help; the NHS offers free help and support for people who want to stop smoking, and there are many other places you can turn to for help.

Ways to help you quit smoking:
- Set a day in advance that you will stop – and tell all your friends, family and workmates so they can support you
- Do it with a friend or colleague. If someone else gives up with you, you will reinforce each other's willpower; maybe you can get some of your workmates to give up at the same time
- Clear the house (and your car, and desk, and anywhere else you keep them) of all your smoking materials – not just cigarettes, but lighters and matches, rolling papers, ashtrays, etc
- Chew on a carrot – not just good for your health anyway (another of your 5-a-day), but it will also give you something to do with your mouth and hands
- Ask your friends not to smoke around you (or at least pretend they're not enjoying it) – people accept this far more readily than they used to

MAN MANUAL 11

- Take things one day at a time, and mark your progress on a chart or calendar
- Keep all the money you've saved somewhere safe – and then treat yourself with it
- Make use of any prescription or non-prescription aids available (your pharmacist or GP can advise you on this); or maybe try alternative therapies like hypnotherapy or acupuncture
- Join a 'stop-smoking' support group for professional advice and support from other people.

> **Did you know?**
> Smokers are at least 50% more likely to have erection problems than non-smokers.

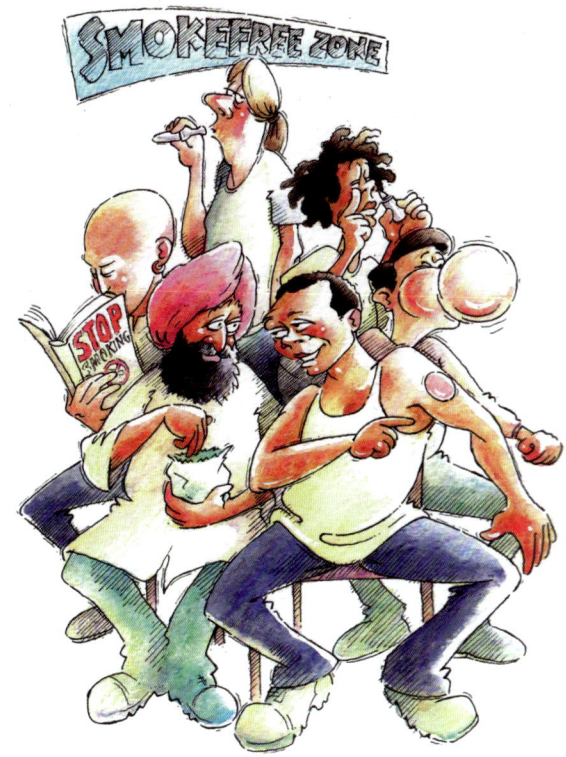

Useful contacts

NHS – Go Smokefree
0800 022 4332
www.smokefree.nhs.uk

Action on Smoking and Health
0207 739 5902
www.ash.org.uk

Quit
0800 00 22 00
www.quit.org.uk

Sensible drinking

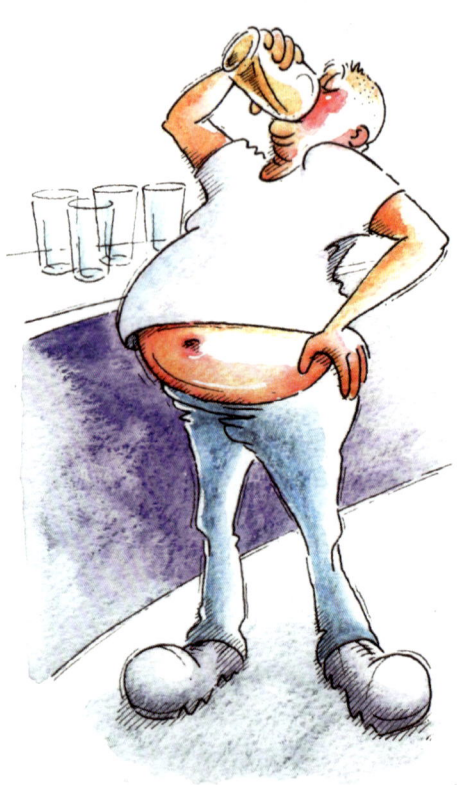

Lower risk drinking means no more than 3 to 4 units a day for men. If you keep to these amounts you will help prevent damaging your health. (if you're not sure what a unit of alcohol is, check out the table Just how heavy is your drinking.)

If you regularly drink more than 35 units a week you might already have experienced problems like feeling tired or depressed, putting on weight, memory loss, sleeping badly and having sexual problems. You could also suffer from high blood pressure. Some people are argumentative if they drink a lot, which can affect their relationships with family and friends.

See www.malehealth.co.uk/drinking

Just how heavy is your drinking?		
Large glass of wine (175 millilitres) 15%	3 units	120 to 170 calories
Small glass of wine (125 millilitres) 12%	1½ units	85 to 120 calories
Bottle of wine (750 millilitres) 12%	9 units	510 to 720 calories
Pint of beer 5%	3 units	180 calories
Pint of beer 3.5%	2 units	160 to 170 calories
Single measure of spirits (25 millilitres) 40%	1 unit	60 to 75 calories

For more information go to **www.drinkaware.co.uk** or call **0800 917 8282**.

Drinking tips

- Walk to the pub to burn off some extra calories on the way
- Drink plenty of water, both during the day and when drinking alcohol
- Try to drink after a meal instead of before – you won't spoil your appetite and you won't feel like drinking so much after your meal
- Try reducing the strength of what you drink. For example, if you normally drink 5% beer, try 3.5% beer instead
- Try to have at least 2 alcohol-free days a week
- A glass of water before your meal may help you both eat and drink less.

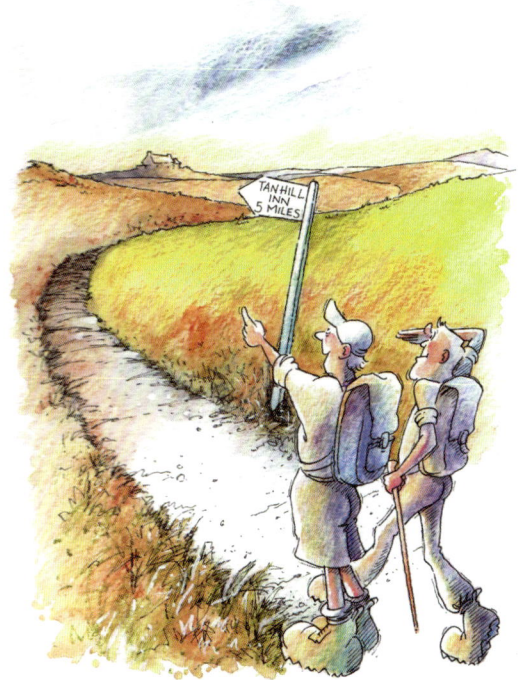

Drugs and substance use

There are many different types of drugs, each with their own facts, issues and risks, too many to cover in this guide. For frank, confidential information from friendly people who are professionally trained to give straight up, unbiased information about drugs, ring Frank on 0800 77 66 00, or check out www.talktofrank.com. The lines are open 24 hours a day, 365 days a year and offer translation services. Both the helpline and website also give confidential information and support for those worried about a friend or family member.

Eyes

Most fish have eyes on each side of their head. This means they can see in two directions at the same time. Sounds a great idea but they still end up in a very big net. Human eyes look ahead and we only wish we had eyes in the back of our heads – would come in hand at times! Poor vision is a major cause of accidents. Eye injuries are a major cause of poor or even loss of vision.

Injury

The surface of the eye is vulnerable to damage by foreign bodies or by irritating substances. Where appropriate, wear protective glasses, goggles or a face shield. Immediate irrigation with lots of water will often wash out foreign bodies and is essential for severe irritants. Foreign bodies may also be removed directly.

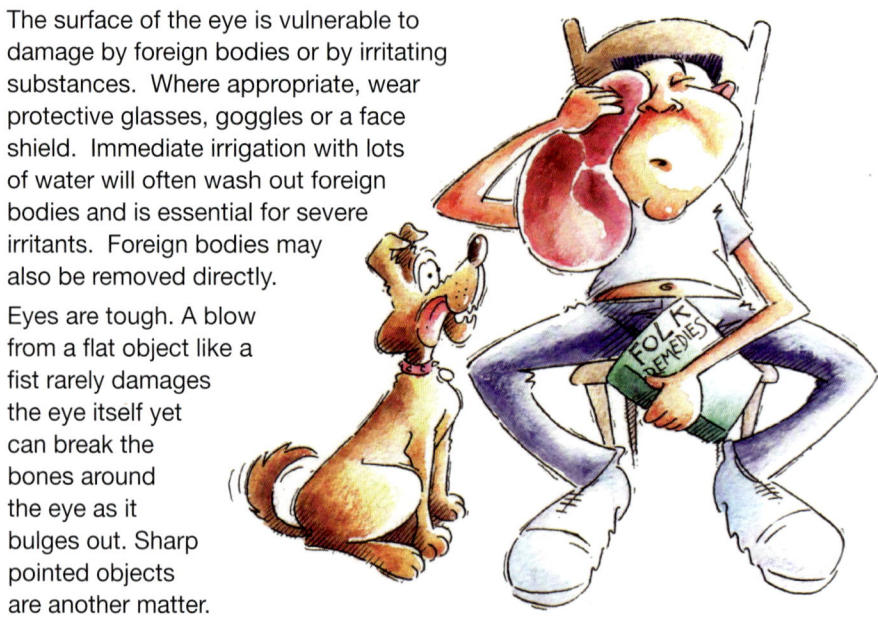

Eyes are tough. A blow from a flat object like a fist rarely damages the eye itself yet can break the bones around the eye as it bulges out. Sharp pointed objects are another matter. Metal splinters from a hammer-strike travel at the speed of sound and can pass right through the front of the eye, damaging the sensitive retina at the back. This can lead to the loss of sight in both eyes even though only one has been injured.

Action point
- Wear the right protective gear when handling tools.

Poor vision

Accidents aren't the only cause of worsening sight.

Infection

Eye infections are common and can cause redness, pain, itchiness and intermittent blurring of vision from pus. Conjunctivitis (infection of the surface of the eye) is catching so use your own towel. Ask your pharmacist for antibiotic drops or cream.

Glaucoma
Caused by pressure building up inside the eye. It is passed down the family so get checked out by an optometrist before it hits you. Some forms of glaucoma cause severe eye pain and halos around lights. These require urgent treatment to prevent permanent blindness.

Impairment of vision
As we age our eyes frequently develop problems. Some people lose distance vision, others lose near vision. For some of us such difficulties are there throughout life and can normally be corrected by the use of glasses or lenses. See an optometrist if you find you are having problems. Cataract is another cause of impaired vision that becomes more common with age. An optometrist can advise on treatment.

Ears

Poor hearing is no joke for anyone.

Noise Induced Hearing Loss creeps up on you. More and more you are asking people to say it again or getting abuse for playing music too loud. Hearing also deteriorates with age: around 42% of over 50 year-olds in the UK have some kind of hearing loss.

Action points
- Wear ear protectors when appropriate
- Let your ears rest after being exposed to unavoidable noise
- See your doctor if your hearing is getting worse.

Action on Hearing Loss offer a hearing test online or via the telephone - **www.actiononhearingloss.org.uk** or call 0844 800 3838

Lug holes blocked?
Wax is a common cause of reduced hearing especially when water gets trapped behind it.
See your GP.
Do not stick anything in your ear. Fuse wire, matchsticks, six inch nails all are bad ideas.

Mouth matters

Men visit their dentist less often than women. It can be difficult to find time to get to a dentist and it's not exactly the first thing you want to do. However, most things that go wrong in your mouth can be prevented. Getting a check-up can avoid a lot of pain and even an unnecessary extraction.

Tooth decay and gum disease

Sugary foods and drinks feed the plaque bacteria that live naturally in the mouth. The bacteria then make acid which attacks the tooth enamel causing tooth decay. The bacteria also irritates the gums which can cause gum disease. Most older people who lose their teeth, do so because of gum disease. Smoking also causes gum disease. Preventing all this is quite simple:

Action points
- Brush your teeth AND GUMS every night and morning with a fluoride toothpaste. And spit but don't rinse to keep the fluoride working
- Try to keep sugary foods and drinks to mealtimes only. Choose healthier snacks between meals such as fruit and vegetables
- Visit a dentist at least once a year.

Mouth cancer

Men are more likely than women to get cancer of the mouth, lips or throat. Most of these cancers are caused by smoking (or chewing tobacco) and excessive alcohol intake. Watch out for:

- Any white or red patches, an ulcer or lump (which may not be painful), which does not go away within two weeks
- Early diagnosis is critical - go and see your doctor or dentist as soon as possible.

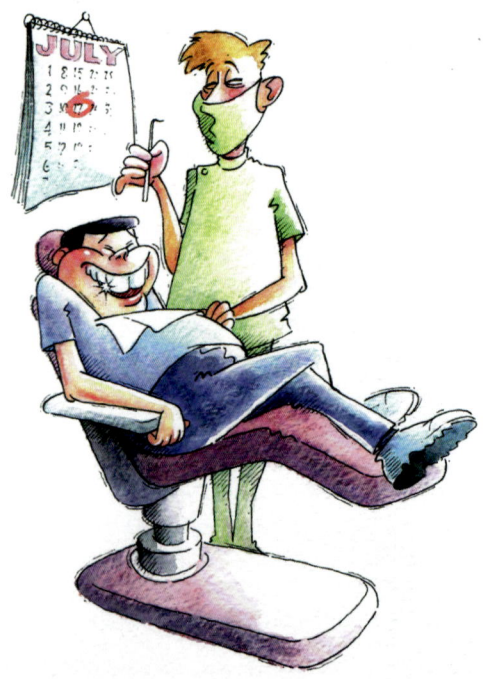

Back pain

If you've ever suffered from a bad back you'll know just how painful and restrictive it can be – and because other people cannot 'see' the pain it tends to get little sympathy. Bad backs are also one the greatest causes of sickness-related absence from work. The good news though is that back pain is rarely serious and the best advice is to keep moving and stay active.

If your job involves lifting heavy objects, sitting at a desk or being immobile for long periods of time, checking your back makes good sense. Chronic back pain can result from bad posture, poor lifting technique or accidental injury.

Being overweight is also a major cause of back problems, not least because it can reduce activity and flexibility, but because it also puts added strain on the muscles, ligaments and bones of the spine. Smoking can also significantly reduce bone strength – which is another good reason for quitting.

Adult bone is constantly being altered and renewed. This needs plenty of calcium. The body can only store this vital mineral in the bone itself, so fresh calcium is needed on a daily basis. The best sources are dairy products such as milk, cheese and yoghurt, but bread is also good as are fish (such as sardines) with edible bones and green leafy vegetables. You should include some of these foods in your meals on a routine basis. Adults should be eating around 700mg of calcium every day.

Bones are not the only cause of back pain. The back is supported by hundreds of different muscles including those that also support the arms, legs and head. These range from enormously strong muscles seen over the back to those inside the body. All of them can be strained or overworked leaving the spine vulnerable to damage – in fact, most back pain comes from injured muscle or tendons rather than the spine itself.

Looking after your back

When standing for long periods
- Head – keep it up and in line with your spine
- Shoulders – relax and pull in your shoulder blades
- Pelvis – keep your hips level while tucking-in your tailbone to line up with your spine
- Knees – keep slightly bent (not locked)
- Feet – share the weight evenly.

When driving
- Head – use a head restraint at all times

- Lower back – adjust the seat (or use a small cushion) to give maximum support, and sit well back without slouching
- Arms – slightly bent
- Legs – adjust the seat for ease of reaching the pedals (while allowing maximum visibility)
- Take a break – when stopped at the lights, relax by taking your hands off the wheel and bending your legs.

When lifting heavy objects
- Keep your back straight and use your legs to take the strain
- Know your limits, if it's a two-man job then don't be a one man bad back. It's not always just weight but also the awkward shape or location of a load that can cause problems

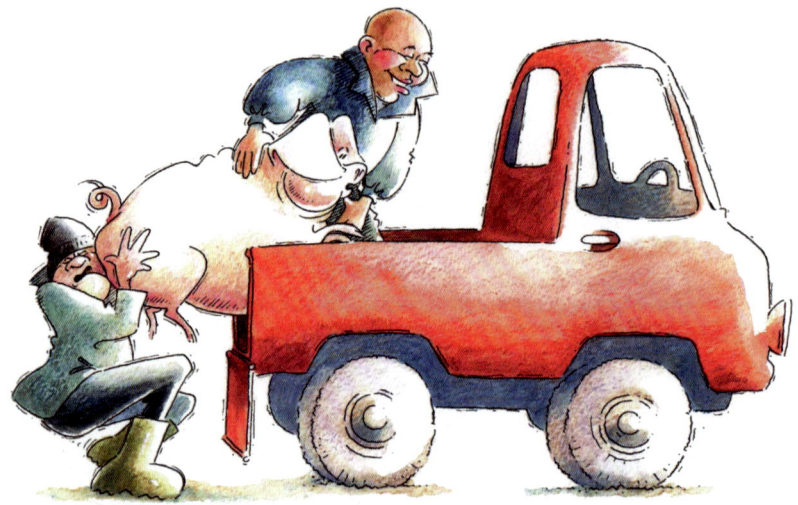

- Make sure you can deal with the shape, clear the area and warn people before you attempt a lift. If the forklifts or trolleys are being used by someone else, wait until they are free – machines are much easier to repair than people.

When using a computer
- VDU – ensure the screen is free from glare and you can clearly see the image (glare can cause headaches)
- Chair – adjust your chair so your eyes are level with the top of the VDU, your forearms are approximately parallel, and your legs can be moved freely with no pressure from the edge of your seat on the backs of your legs and knees (a footrest may be helpful); if you already have a bad back, a chair with adjustable lumbar support can be particularly helpful

- Keyboard – adjust the keyboard so you can rest your hands and wrists in front of the keyboard, and keep your wrists straight while typing (poor wrist posture can also lead to RSI or carpal tunnel syndrome – both extremely painful and debilitating)
- Mouse – again adjust the mouse so it is within easy reach and can be used with the wrist straight while supporting your forearm on the desk
- Take short regular breaks – don't sit in the same position for too long, make sure you stretch your legs and change your posture.

Absent from work with back pain

If you are away from work for prolonged periods with back pain, it is important that you stay in regular contact with your employer to make them aware of your situation, to be kept informed about developments at work and to discuss what adjustments might be needed once you are ready to return.

Discuss your needs with your employer and occupational health provider and try to suggest any practical workplace adaptations or alterations which might help you to cope while you return to full-time working. If there is no occupational health provider available, your GP or safety representative may be able to discuss possible work adjustments. Returning to work can be part of your recovery from back pain.

Dealing with a period of back pain and returning to work

It is important to stay at work if you can, as this helps you to keep active and recover from the pain. If you have a lot of lifting or other risk factors in your job, talk to your supervisor or boss and tell them about tasks that will be difficult to begin with initially.

A gentle return to full activity is better than weeks of lying in bed with a door under the mattress (in fact, lying flat in a bed for three weeks only makes things worse as it weakens the supporting muscles). Traction (putting huge weights on the legs) belongs in a museum of horrors – it would take a double-decker bus to counter the strength of the back muscles!

If you are suffering from a bad back, when you lie down, try to reduce the pressure on the spine by lying sideways with the legs slightly bent and a cushion between them. Tension is part of the problem, so getting someone to give you a gentle back massage can work wonders. Don't stay in the same position too long; although movement may be painful, it is best to roll over and stand up and walk around. A mix of non-steroidal anti-inflammatory medicines (such as ibuprofen) along with paracetamol can help enormously – always use them according to the instructions on the packet. Warm towels alternated with cool compresses can help relax muscles (warm) and reduce inflammation (cool). As the pain subsides try to regain normal activity but avoid lifting or straining.

Sexually transmitted infections (STIs)

Sexually transmitted infections (STIs) can infect at any age, whether straight or gay, in a long-term relationship or with a casual partner. Symptoms don't always show up immediately, so the infection could be recent or from a long time ago. Some STIs such as chlamydia may be more or less symptom-free but can still cause long-term damage.

The best way to prevent sexually transmitted infections is to practise safer sex. Use a condom whenever you have sex, unless of course you're trying to conceive or are in a monogamous long-term relationship where both parties are certain that they are infection-free. Some infections such as hepatitis B can also be transmitted by sharing needles, razor blades or even a toothbrush.

If you have had unsafe sex or are at all worried, you can have a confidential check-up, and treatment if needed, at a genitourinary medicine (GUM) or STI clinic.

Although extra lubrication is sometimes needed, do not use oil-based lubricants such as petroleum jelly or baby oil with condoms, as they will damage the condom (as can lipstick!). There are water-based lubricants available, but if you are not sure, ask your chemist – they will not be embarrassed to give you advice.

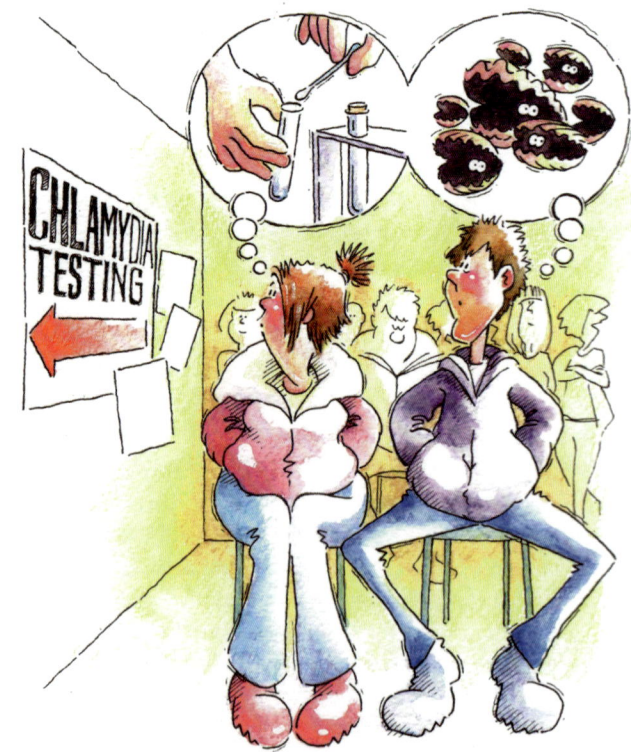

Erectile dysfunction (ED, impotence)

At least one in 10 British men have had some sort of erection problems at some stage in their lives and around one man in 20 has permanent erection problems. This is not helped by most men not wanting to talk about these problems, despite the fact that virtually all of them can be sorted out with simple treatments.

> It is very important to find out what is causing the problem as it may be linked to diabetes or high blood pressure.

At one time, what a man was thinking about was considered the major factor for erection problems. We now know that around one-third of all cases will be due to psychological issues and can often respond well to non-clinical treatments such as sex counselling.

Normally, if you have erections at any time other than during attempted intercourse you have a psychological rather than physical problem. Getting an erection during television programmes, sexy videos or self-masturbation is a good sign, although it is not a 100% test.

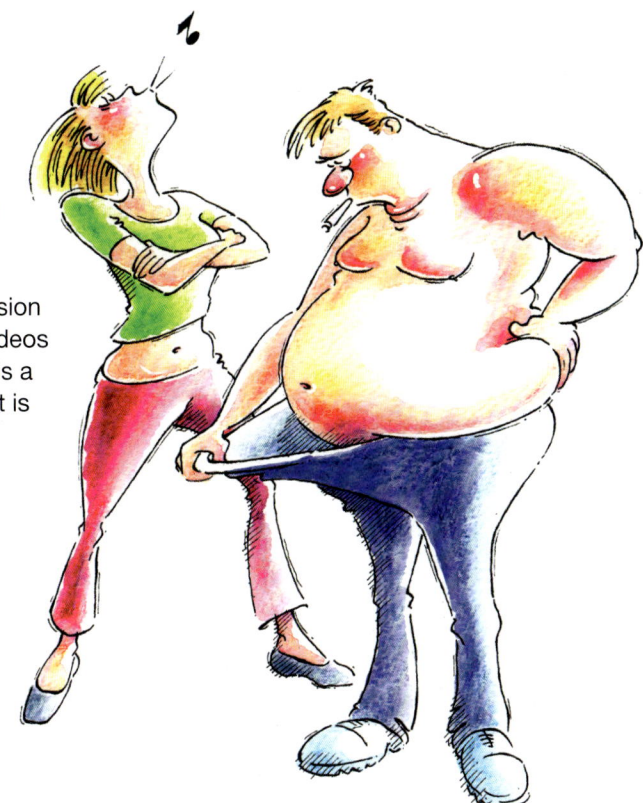

Prostate problems

Only men have a prostate gland. It's round and about the size of a golf ball. It is in the pelvis, against the base of the bladder. The prostate surrounds the urethra – the tube that runs from your bladder inside your penis to the outside (you urinate through it). Imagine the prostate as a fat rubber washer around a bit of tubing. It grows to adult size during puberty. In most men it also begins to grow again in early middle age, which can cause problems which are quite common.

There are two possible causes of an enlarged prostate: benign prostate hyperplasia (BPH) – a benign (non-cancerous) enlargement of the prostate gland common in men over 50 – and prostate cancer. The symptoms are very similar and are usually related to problems urinating, such as the following.

- A constant need to urinate, especially at night
- Rushing to the toilet
- Difficulty starting to urinate
- Difficulty urinating
- Taking a long time urinating
- Having a weak flow of urine
- Feeling that your bladder has not emptied properly
- Dribbling after you've finished urinating
- Pain or discomfort when urinating.

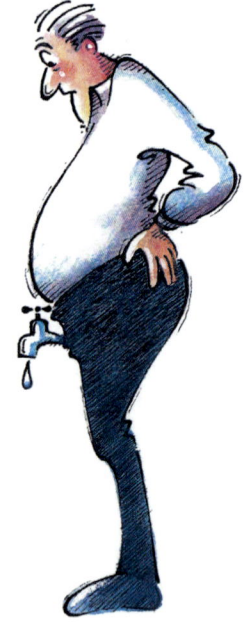

Other symptoms can include the following:

- Lower back pain
- Pain in your pelvis, hips or thighs
- Erection problems
- Blood in the urine – this is rare
- Pain when you ejaculate
- Pain in your penis or testicles.

It is important that you know that any of these symptoms can also be caused by problems which are nothing to do with prostate cancer. If you are concerned about any symptoms that you have, visit your doctor.

Enlarged prostate (BPH)

BPH rarely causes symptoms before the age of 40, but more than half of men in their sixties and as many as 90% in their seventies and eighties have some symptoms of BPH.

As the prostate enlarges, tissue layers surrounding it prevents it from growing evenly, and pressure then squashes the urethra like a clamp on a garden hose. As a result, the bladder wall becomes thicker and irritated, shrinking even when it contains small amounts of urine, causing you to urinate more often. The bladder will eventually weaken and lose the ability to empty itself, trapping urine inside. The urethra becoming narrower and the bladder not emptying completely cause many of the problems linked with BPH. Some men with very enlarged prostates might not suffer while others with less-enlarged prostates can have more problems.

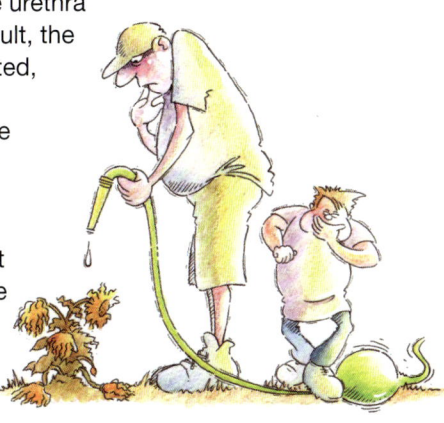

The problem can be treated with drugs or by surgically removing the enlarged part of the prostate. There is a small risk that either treatment may cause impotence (being unable to get and keep an erection). You can speak to your doctor about this.

Prostate cancer

Older men of African or Caribbean origin are at high risk of getting prostate cancer. Men who have had a close male blood relative, especially a brother, with prostate cancer also seem to have an increased risk of getting it.

The Western diet of highly refined food with a high animal fat content also seems to increase the risk of developing prostate cancer. There is no firm evidence of how to reduce the risk of prostate cancer. We do know that having a healthy diet with more fruit and vegetables, less red meat and more fish is good for reducing the risks of other cancers, heart disease and possibly prostate cancer.

It is important to be clear – not all men get symptoms that show they have prostate cancer. In the men that do, not all men have exactly the same symptoms. You do not have to have all the symptoms listed to have prostate cancer.

Prostate cancer is treated in several different ways, which can depend on how aggressive the cancer is, whether it has spread elsewhere in your body and how old you are. Your general state of health may also make a difference.

You can speak to your doctor about your options.

> You may be able to reduce your risk with the occasional Bloody Mary, preferably with more tomato juice than vodka. Tomatoes are said to protect you.

For more information go to **www.yourprostate.eu**

Bowel cancer

What is bowel cancer?
Bowel cancer is a disease of the large bowel (colon) or rectum. It is also sometimes called colorectal or colon cancer.

- It is the second largest cause of cancer deaths in the UK
- In 2006 there were over 30,000 new cases of bowel cancer in England and over 14,000 deaths
- Around one in 20 people will get bowel cancer at some point in their life.

Causes of bowel cancer

The definite cause of bowel cancer is still a mystery. But we know some things do increase your risk. Your risk is higher if:

- You eat lots of junk food, fat and sugar and not enough fibre
- You eat lots of burnt food
- Someone in your close family had bowel cancer
- You don't exercise
- You're overweight
- You smoke tobacco.

The good news is you can reduce your risk, even if bowel cancer is in the family.

- Reduce fats and sugars in your diet and eat more fruit, vegetables and fibre
- Keep your weight under control
- Discuss your family history with your doctor
- Quit smoking.

Better sooner than later

Being 'bowel aware' is the name of the game. Guts play up at the best of times but there are some warning signs that you shouldn't ignore. Symptoms that might be bowel cancer include:

- A *persistent* change in normal bowel habit, such as going more often and diarrhoea, especially if you are also bleeding from your bottom
- Bleeding from the bottom without any reason
- A lump in your tummy or back passage felt by your doctor
- Pain that affects your appetite
- Unexplained iron deficiency
- Unexplained weight loss
- Unexplained extreme tiredness.

If you have any of these symptoms for four weeks you should go and see your GP, but please remember that most of these symptoms will not be cancer.

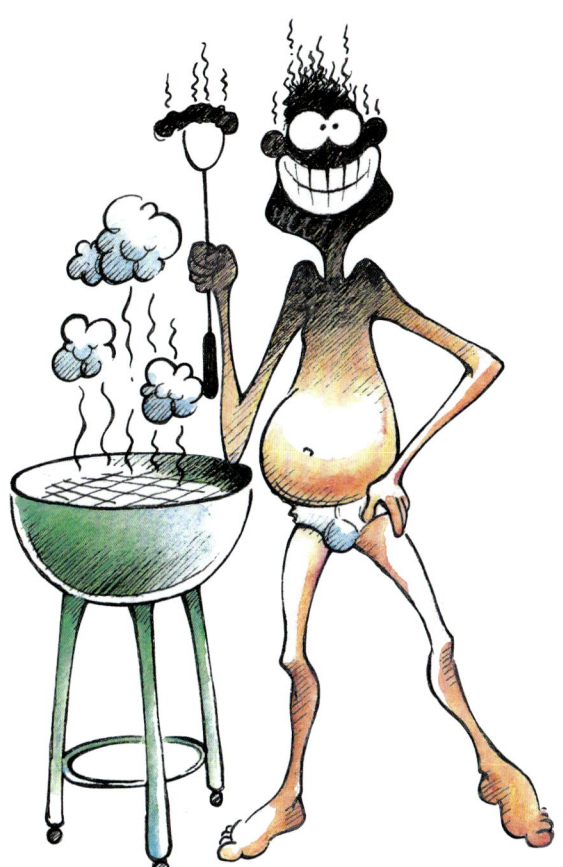

Getting it sorted

If you do have bowel cancer, treatment will depend on where the cancer is, whether it has spread and your general health. Surgery is the main form of treatment, but more doctors are combining it with chemotherapy and radiotherapy.

Useful contacts

NHS Cancer Screening Programmes
www.cancerscreening.nhs.uk

Beating Bowel Cancer
www.beatingbowelcancer.org

Bowel Cancer UK
Helpline: 0800 8 40 35 40
www.bowelcanceruk.org.uk

Cancer Research UK
0808 800 4040
www.cancerhelp.org.uk

Macmillan
Free telephone help line
0808 808 00 00
www.macmillan.org.uk

Skin cancer

"We need to understand that sun cream is not just for when you are on holiday."

The sun damages your skin by its ultraviolet radiation (UV). (Tanning is a sign that damaged skin is trying to protect itself from the sun's ultraviolet rays.) As you might expect, farmers suffer skin cancer more than people with indoor jobs.

There are basically two types of skin cancer. Non-melanoma is the most common form. Watch out for:

- A new growth or sore that does not heal within four weeks
- A spot or sore that continues to itch, hurt, crust, scab or bleed
- Constant skin ulcers that are not explained by other causes.

These are commonly found on the forehead and on the tip of the chin, nose or ears; i.e. the exposed bits.

Malignant melanoma is the more serious form of skin cancer. Although it is much less common, it is on the increase. It most often appears as a changing mole or freckle. Watch out for:

- Size: bigger than the butt end of a pencil (more than 6mm/quarter inch diameter)
- Colour variety: shades of tan, brown or black and sometimes red, blue or white
- Shape: ragged or scalloped edge and one half unlike the other
- Itchiness
- Bleeding
- Look at your moles and watch out for changes in them.

Many skin changes are harmless but a quick check with your doctor or pharmacist can save your skin.

Sun Smart Tips
- If possible, seek shade when the sun is strong
- Wear a t-shirt and long shorts made from closely woven fabric
- Slap on a hat. A big hat (that covers ears, neck and nose!)
- Slop on sunscreen with SPF 15+ every 2 hours
- Wear sunglasses to protect your eyes.

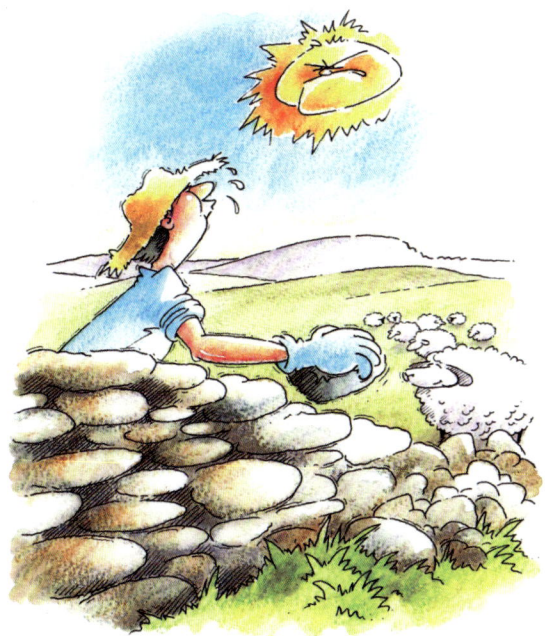

Sunscreens and smokescreens

People get confused over sunscreens and can damage their skin by choosing the wrong sunscreen for them or not using enough.

Read your suncreen label and make sure it has both an SPF and a star rating. The SPF or Sun Protection Factor tells you how much protection you are getting from UVB rays.

The star *** rating shows the level of protection against UVA rays. Try to buy a sunscreen that is at least SPF 15+ and has a 4 star rating.

Remember! Sunscreen offers some protection, but use it with cover-up clothing.

Not a lot of people know this
- Skin cancer is the most common cancer in the UK and not just in women
- Your lifetime risk as a man of developing skin cancer is one in eight
- Even cloudy days can deliver 90% of the dangerous UV rays
- Some football shirts are so thin they let almost all the sunshine through
- Skin damage builds up under the skin just like rust under bodywork paint and cancome back to haunt you in later years
- Virtually all the risk comes from the sun ... so cover up!

Testicular cancer

Testicular problems are quite rare, and testicular cancer is the most serious. It represents only 1% of all cancers in men, but it is the single biggest cause of cancer-related death in men aged between 18 and 35.

Symptoms of testicular cancer
- A lump on one testicle
- Pain and tenderness in either testicle
- Discharge (pus or smelly goo) from the penis
- Blood in the sperm when you ejaculate
- A build-up of fluid inside the testicular sac (scrotum)
- A heavy dragging feeling in the groin or scrotum
- An increase in the size of a testicle
- An enlargement of the breasts, with or without tenderness.

Preventing testicular cancer

For once, men are positively encouraged to check themselves, but this time to do more than just 'check they're still there'. Self-examination is the name of the game. Check your testicles every month in the following ways.

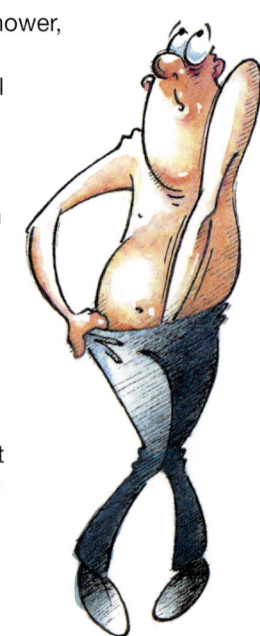

- Do it lying in a warm bath or while having a long shower, as this makes the skin of the scrotum softer
- Hold the scrotum in the palm of your hand and feel the difference between the testicles. You will very probably feel that one is larger and lying lower, which is completely normal
- Examine each one in turn, and then compare them with each other. Use both hands and gently roll each testicle between your thumb and forefinger. Check for any lumps or swellings as they should both be smooth. Remember that the duct carrying sperm to the penis, the epididymis, normally feels bumpy. It lies along the top and back of the testis.

Checking your testicles too often can actually make it more difficult to notice any difference and may cause unnecessary worry.

When health problems develop

Catching problems early

Almost all health problems can be more easily and successfully treated the earlier they are caught. Apart from consulting your GP as soon as symptoms develop, check-ups and screening programmes provided by the NHS or the workplace can be beneficial.

Visiting your GP

OK, we all know men tend to be more reluctant to consult a GP than women, but if you are serious about improving your health and living a longer and healthier life, you really need to change this attitude. Not only can your GP provide good advice on a whole range of health related matters, GPs are also best placed to know what to do once you develop a health problem.

Just remember: you may have read this 'quick manual' to your body, but your GP has the full manual and spent many years studying it. By analogy, almost anyone can do a quick oil change or top-up the water level on their car, but even the most gifted amateur would still be wise to use a qualified mechanic for a major job like rebuilding a gearbox.

Returning to work

For a long time, when people developed health problems the standard approach was to visit their GP for a sick note and then stay off work until they felt better. Nowadays, attitudes to health and work have changed and it has become widely recognised that work is beneficial to health and being workless is bad for health. Indeed no one is 100% fit – and prolonged absences from work on sick leave can actually make some health problems worse.

Speak to your GP and discuss the timing for a return to work. Your employer can help if you need any adjustments to help you return to work. These could be:

- Reduced hours – building up the hours to full time over a reasonable period
- Modified duties – if your normal job is physically demanding your employer may be able to offer you a more sedentary role
- Workplace adjustments – this includes appropriate seating if your work involves sitting for prolonged periods
- Time off work to attend hospital or physiotherapy appointments.

Many employers also offer some form of occupational health provision for their staff. If this is available, you should make use of it as it can often enable you to receive treatment more quickly than you could by going through the NHS.

Getting the best from the NHS

Don't get caught in the web

Buying drugs from illegal internet sites is potentially very dangerous. Almost all such drugs are at best fake and useless, at worst harmful. You may also have your credit card details stolen as well. More important is the danger of not getting a medical diagnosis. Erection problems won't kill you but linked diabetes or high blood pressure most certainly can. You should speak your doctor or chemist about this first.

More than ever before, the NHS has a range of services that offer convenient options that allow you to get the right treatment at the right time, and at the right place. These services can make life a lot easier so visit www.nhsdirect.nhs.uk or phone 0845 4647.

Pharmacists: more than just blue bottles

Pharmacists are highly-qualified professionals providing advice on the use and selection of prescription and over-the-counter (OTC) medicines. They can give advice on how to manage small problems and common conditions. This includes lifestyle advice about eating habits, exercise and stopping smoking, but they will also tell you where you can get further advice.

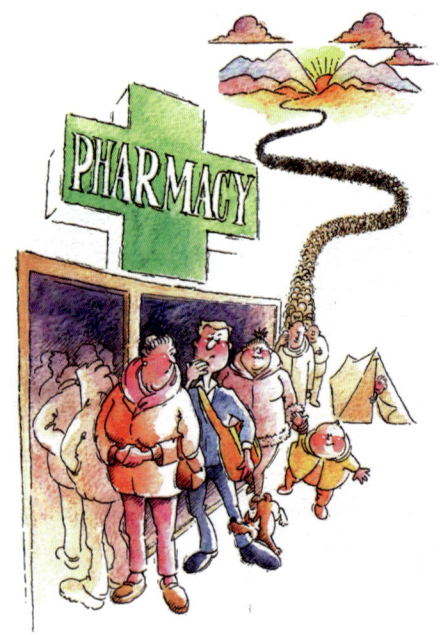

NHS Walk-in Centres: a step in the right direction

Highly qualified NHS nurses offer a range of convenient and free services, with no need to make an appointment. They also offer good advice, look after minor illnesses and injuries, provide prescriptions and even provide emergency contraception. Look out for the centres in railway stations, shopping centres or on the high street. They normally open from 7am until 10pm, Monday to Friday, and 9am to 10pm, Saturday and Sunday.

NHS Direct: direct and to the point

NHS Direct provides 24-hour confidential health advice and information. Phone 0845 4647 or visit NHS Direct Online at **www.nhsdirect.nhs.uk**. Why not try NHS Direct Interactive on digital satellite TV?

Doctors' surgeries

Doctors are often available from around 8.30am to 6pm (or later). Calling at other times will put you in touch with an out-of-hours system. It's always best to see your own doctor if possible, so unless your problem is urgent and cannot wait, you should make an appointment to be seen by your normal doctor. Practices now often offer a huge range of services such as minor surgery, skincare, chiropody and even diabetic clinics.

Getting the best from your doctor

If you don't turn up for an appointment you can cause huge frustration, especially because you haven't had any medical attention. You should:

- Write down your symptoms before you see your doctor. It's extremely easy to forget the most important things during the examination. Doctors will spot important clues about a problem by asking questions such as: When did the problem start and how did it feel? Did anyone else suffer as well? Has this ever happened before? What have you done about it so far? Are you taking any medicine for it?
- Ask questions, and don't be afraid to ask your doctor to give more information or make something clear that you don't understand. Asking them to write it down for you is a good idea
- Get to the point – if you have a lump or bump say so. Time is limited so there is a real danger of you coming out with a prescription for a sore nose when you might need a serious problem sorted
- Have your prescription explained, and ask whether you can buy any medicines from your chemist. Make sure you know what each medicine is for. Some medicines clash badly with alcohol.

Dentists

You will have to pay for dental check-ups and treatment unless you are at school, are pregnant or receive certain benefits. To find an NHS dentist in your area, go to **www.nhs.uk**.

Accident and emergency

Accident and emergency departments treat serious accidents or life-threatening illnesses such as heart attacks or medical conditions which suddenly become worse. They are open 24 hours a day all year, and are often used by people who should really see their own doctor or a pharmacist. You should be prepared to wait if there are people more seriously ill than you.

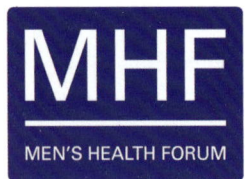

Cash or Cheque Donations Form

I would like to support the work of Men's Health Forum and enclose a donation of £ . . . .

Name: . . . .

Address: . . . .

. . . .

. . . .

Postcode: . . . .

E-mail: . . . .

Signature: . . . .

Date: . . . .

By ticking the box below we can reclaim 28p in tax for every pound you donate:

Gift aid it!

☐ Yes! Please treat all donations I make to Men's Health Forum from this date forward as Gift Aid donations. I confirm I am a UK tax payer and I pay an amount of UK income or capital gains tax at least equal to the tax that Men's Health Forum will reclaim on my donations in the tax year. Please remember to notify us if your circumstances change and you no longer pay an amount of tax equal to the tax we will reclaim.

Thank you so much for your support.

Please return your completed form to:
Men's Health Forum,
32-36 Loman Street, London SE1 0EH

Please make a donation to the Men's Health Forum

The Men's Health Forum works towards improving the quality of life for men and boys among vulnerable and at-risk populations in England and Wales. We achieve this goal by providing free self-help information and resources tailored to the needs of boys and men as well as developing local community health interventions. **All our resources and services are free of advertising and influence.** Please help us keep it that way. **We need your support to continue our independent work.** For every £1 donated, we spend:

1. 30p to fill the gap in medical knowledge by conducting unique men's health specific research

2. 30p to produce independent, free-of-advertising men's health resources such as this men's health manual

3. 30p to build innovative health education programs and health promotion campaigns in the communities across England and Wales

4. And no more than 10p on ongoing expenses to support the general operations

Donations, small or large, are very much appreciated. **Please make a donation today to keep our mission strong.**